BLOOD TYPE

B-NEGATIVE

DIET BOOK

"60 Simple and Delicious Recipes for Lifelong Health and Weight Loss"

Dayna G. Murphy

GAIN ACCESS TO OTHER BLOOD TYPE BOOKS BY ME

Table of Contents

INTRODUCTION

Within the vibrant workplace filled with a variety of personalities, a group of coworkers who were all Blood Type B negative were gradually changing. Joined by their shared experience, they set out to investigate the advantages of modifying their diets to correspond with their blood type. As they started eating the suggested meals, good things started to happen.

Sarah, who used to have afternoon energy slumps, experienced renewed energy by making protein-rich food choices. Including lean proteins and healthy carbohydrates gave her a steady energy boost that made it easy for her to get through the workday.

John, who is well-known for having sensitive digestive systems, discovered comfort by steering clear of troublesome proteins and paying attention to specific carbohydrates. A blood type-appropriate diet helped him feel less bloated and uncomfortable, which improved his concentration.

Amy, a fitness enthusiast, chose foods that complemented her blood type to enhance her workout performance. She experienced increased muscle recovery and stamina throughout her intensive exercise sessions after choosing the appropriate combination of nutrients.

Talks centered around blood type-appropriate snacks and inventive lunch ideas in the office kitchen. Working together, colleagues shared ideas and found delicious ways to eat well while following their individual diet plans.

The good changes were noticeable as the weeks went by. The once worn-out and lethargic group had transformed into a lively and enthusiastic team, and they credited their improved health to the straightforward but significant decision to eat according to their blood type. The workplace culture changed to one of health consciousness, demonstrating that sometimes even a minor change in nutrition can have a big impact on general wellbeing.

CHAPTER 1

Knowing Your Blood Types

The presence or lack of particular antigens on the surface of red blood cells determines blood type. Blood is divided into four primary types according to the ABO blood group system: A, B, AB, and O. Furthermore, blood is classified as positive (+) or negative (-) based on the Rh factor. Eight major blood types are produced as a result, Type B Negative being one of them.

The genetic makeup that each blood type inherits from its parents determines its individuality. The interaction of Rh and ABO factors influences several physiological characteristics, including compatibility for blood transfusions, susceptibility to specific illnesses, and, surprisingly, nutritional requirements.

Blood Type Is Important for Diet

According to research, blood type may influence how the body responds to certain foods. A naturopathic physician, established the Blood Type Diet, which places special emphasis on this notion. This notion suggests that people with Type B Negative blood could gain from following a diet that is compatible with their blood type.

1. Maximizing Metabolism and Digestion: Blood type B antigens affect stomach acid production and digestive enzyme levels. Knowing these things can help you choose foods that promote healthy metabolism and digestion.

2. Absorption of Nutrients: Different blood types may require different amounts of nutrients. Adapting the diet to the needs of individuals with Type B Negative blood can improve the body's ability to absorb vital vitamins and minerals, which can benefit general health.

3. Inflammation and Immunity: According to the Blood Type Diet, people with different blood types may be more or less sensitive to particular foods, which can have an impact on immune system function and inflammation levels. This involves choosing foods that are less likely to cause inflammation if you are Type B Negative.

4. Weight management: Blood type diet proponents contend that following one's blood type when eating can help with weight management. Knowing how Type B Negative blood responds to various food categories might help you reach and stay at a healthy weight.

5. Energy Levels and Mental Clarity: Maintaining consistent energy levels and mental clarity can be facilitated by a healthy diet. The goal of adjusting food choices to the special requirements of Type B Negative blood is to supply the energy required for maximum everyday performance.

Many people find value in knowing their blood type and choosing foods that suit it, even if the scientific evidence behind the Blood Type Diet is still up for debate. It's critical to approach this idea with an open mind, taking into account individual differences and seeking the assistance of healthcare professionals for tailored guidance.

CHAPTER 2

Unveiling Blood Type B Negative

Features of Blood Type B Negative

1. Antibodies and Antigens:

- B antigens are present on the surface of red blood cells and anti-A antibodies are present in plasma in people with B negative blood type.
- The absence of the Rh antigen is shown by the Rh factor being negative.

2. Genetic Transmission:

- When the B gene is passed down without the presence of the A gene from both parents, the result is the B negative blood type.

3. Enzymes for Digestion:

- It is thought that those with type B personalities create more amylase, an enzyme that facilitates the breakdown of carbohydrates.

4. Response of the Immune System:

- It is thought that people with Type B negative immune systems adapt well to challenges and may offer a strong resistance against illnesses.

5. Flexibility:

Blood types that are B negative are known for their flexibility and adaptability. Supporters of the Blood Type Diet speculate that people of this blood type could be better able to adjust to dietary modifications.

6. Possible Irregularities:

- People who test negative for type B may be more sensitive to some foods, and the Blood Type Diet advises staying away from particular foods that may cause inflammation and digestive problems.

7. Tendency for Balance:

- It is thought that people with Type B Negative blood types are more balanced in many areas of life, such as stress reduction and general wellbeing.

Health Issues for People Who Are Type B Negative

1. The Dietary Guidelines:

- People who test negative for type B are frequently told to concentrate on eating a varied, well-balanced diet that includes foods like lean protein, green veggies, and some grains.

- Avoiding particular items that the Blood Type Diet advises might be less suitable with Type B Negative blood is one of the recommendations.

2. Gastrointestinal health:

- For those who are Type B Negative, maintaining digestive health is essential because it has been believed that blood type influences digestive enzymes. This entails selecting meals that promote effective nutrient absorption and digestion.

3. Controlling Inflammation:

- According to certain Blood Type Diet proponents, people with Type B Negative blood may be more vulnerable to inflammation brought on by particular foods. Thus, emphasis is placed on controlling inflammation by dietary decisions.

4. Physical Activity and Stress Reduction:

- For general health, it is advised to incorporate regular exercise that is customized to each individual's tastes.
- Since stress can affect one's immune system and overall health, stress management strategies are crucial.

5. Regular Health Check-ups:

- Regular check-ups are necessary to monitor blood pressure, cholesterol, and other important health markers, regardless of blood type.

6. Individual Variations:

- It's important to understand that there are individual differences and that different B Negative blood types will have different health concerns. Professionals in healthcare can provide crucial personalized health advice.

CHAPTER 3

The Science Behind the B Negative Blood Type Diet

Blood Type's Genetic Basis

The genes that determine whether antigens are present on the surface of red blood cells or not are inherited from our parents and constitute the genetic basis of blood type. Three primary alleles are involved in the most popular and extensively used blood type system, the ABO blood group system: A, B, and O. The four main blood types—A, B, AB, and O—are made up of these allele combinations.

1. Allele Combinations:

- A person's blood type is determined by the combination of one allele inherited from each parent.

- Blood type AB people have both A and B antigens, blood type O people have neither A nor B antigens, and blood type A people have A antigens and blood type B people have B antigens.

2. Factor Rh:

- Rh-positive or Rh-negative blood is determined by the Rh factor, another crucial aspect of blood type.

- Blood types (such as A+, B-, and AB+) are further classified based on the presence or lack of the Rh antigen (+).

3. Several Gene Loci:

- Many gene loci are involved in blood type inheritance, which adds to the variety of blood types found in a given community.

4. Mendelian Heredity:

- Mendelian principles govern the inheritance of blood types, whereby the combination of parental alleles determines the blood type inherited by the offspring.

The Effects of Blood Type on Metabolism and Digestion

A naturopathic physician promoted the Blood Type Diet, which postulates that a person's blood type affects how their body metabolizes nutrients and digests food. Advocates of this notion contend that knowledge of these factors might direct people toward the healthiest food options, despite the fact that it is debatable and has no scientific backing. This is a broad summary:

1. Type B Blood and Enzymes for Digestion:

- The Blood Type Diet states that those with Type B blood may have larger quantities of the enzyme amylase, which helps with the breakdown of carbohydrates. This points to a possible adaptation to a range of carbohydrate-rich diets.

2. Blood Type B and Protein:

- For Type B individuals, the diet suggests emphasizing a balanced protein intake, with a focus on lean sources like fish and chicken. It advises staying away from specific proteins that might not mix well with Type B blood.

3. Type of Blood and Metabolism:

- According to the diet theory, a person's blood type can determine which foods help or hinder their ability to metabolize energy. A balance of proteins, veggies, and particular grains is frequently advised for Type B individuals.

4. The inflammatory reaction:

- Blood type diet proponents assert that people with Type B blood may be more vulnerable to inflammation brought on by particular foods. Therefore, the diet advises against the consumption of certain items to manage inflammation.

5. Individual Variations:

It is important to remember that, regardless of blood type, individual differences in genetics, lifestyle, and health conditions can have a significant impact on how the body reacts to various diets.

CHAPTER 4

Foods to Embrace

Options High in Protein for Type B Negative

1. Lean Meats:

- Due to their lean protein content, skinless poultry like chicken and turkey is frequently advised for those with Type B Negative blood.

- Mutton or lamb cuts that are lean may also be good choices.

2. Fish:

- Omega-3 fatty acids are abundant in fatty fish, such as cod, mackerel, and salmon, and they also supply vital proteins.

- Other possibilities that fit the dietary preferences of Type B Negative people are halibut and trout.

3. Dairy products:

- To satisfy their protein requirements, those who are Type B Negative can include dairy products including yogurt, low-fat or skim milk, and some cheeses in their diet.

- Some people might prefer the milk products made from goats over those made from cows.

4. Eggs:

- Especially eggs from omega-3 enriched or free-range sources, eggs are a diverse source of protein that can be consumed by those who have Type B negative blood.

5. Proteins for Vegetarians:

- For plant-based protein, you can include tempeh and tofu, which offer options for people who want or eat a vegetarian or vegan diet.
- Legumes that are high in fiber and protein include black beans and lentils.

Advantageous Carbohydrates

1. Complete Grains:

- Whole grains like quinoa, millet, and oats can be included in a diet that is balanced for people who are Type B Negative.
- Refined white rice should not be used instead of brown or basmati rice.

2. Grain Sprouted:

- Some people believe that sprouted grains, like Ezekiel bread or sprouted wheat bread, are easier to digest and can be incorporated into a diet.

3. Sweet potatoes:

- Sweet potatoes are a wholesome source of carbohydrates that also include vitamins, minerals, and fiber.
- They provide a more healthful option than regular potatoes.

4. Legumes:

- Lentils and chickpeas are high-quality sources of carbohydrates that are also reasonably high in fiber and protein.
- Chickpea-based hummus is a delicious and nourishing side dish.

Produce and Fruits that Promote B-Negative Health

1. Berries:

- Antioxidant-rich blueberries, strawberries, and raspberries may be good for your general health.
- These fruits can be enjoyed as snacks, added to smoothies, or incorporated into salads.

2. Leafy Greens:

- Spinach, kale, and Swiss chard are nutrient-dense leafy greens that provide essential vitamins and minerals.
- They can be used in salads, sautés, or green smoothies.

3. Broccoli and Cauliflower:

- These cruciferous vegetables are high in fiber and offer a variety of vitamins and minerals.
- They can be steamed, roasted, or included in stir-fries.

4. Pineapple and Papaya:

- These tropical fruits provide natural sweetness along with digestive enzymes.
- Pineapple and papaya can be enjoyed fresh or added to fruit salads.

5. Avocado:

- Avocado is a nutrient-dense fruit that is rich in healthy fats, fiber, and various vitamins.
- It can be sliced on toast, added to salads, or blended into a creamy dressing.

CHAPTER 5

Foods to Limit or Avoid

Proteins That Cause Issues for Those Who Are Type B Negative

1. Chicken:

- Chicken is one protein source that Type B Negative people may want to minimize, according to the Blood Type Diet. The reasoning behind this is that people with this blood type might not be able to tolerate all of the lectins present in chicken.

2. Warm wheat:

- Even though buckwheat is a whole grain, those with Type B Negative blood are advised to avoid it or consume it in moderation. According to the notion, some of the ingredients in buckwheat might not mix well with the digestive traits of Type B people.

3. Shellfish:

- People who test negative for Type B negativity are advised against eating some shellfish, including crab and shrimp. According to the notion, people with this blood type might not be able to digest these proteins as quickly.

4. Pork:

- It's common advice for people who are Type B Negative to reduce their intake of pork and pork-derived items in their diet. The logic stems from the theory that certain of the proteins in pork could not be as suitable with this blood type's digestive tract.

5. Meats that have been processed:

- Because of possible additives and preservatives that could not be in line with the blood type's recommended diet, processed meats, such as sausages and bacon, are normally avoided by people with Type B Negative blood.

Carbohydrates You Should Use Carefully

1. Products Made of Wheat:

- Individuals with Type B Negative blood are often recommended to avoid or consume wheat and wheat-based items (mainly breads and pastas) in moderation. According to the Blood Type Diet, some wheat lectins might not be well-tolerated.

2. Corn:

- People who are Type B Negative are advised against eating corn and corn products. According to the notion, people with this blood type may be adversely affected by the lectins included in corn.

3. Tomatoes:

- Even though tomatoes are a common vegetable, people who are Type B Negative are advised to limit their intake according to the Blood Type Diet. It implies that some tomato ingredients might not be as friendly to people with this blood type's digestive systems.

4. Soy-Based Products:

- People with Type B Negative blood are advised to consume soy products, such as tofu and soy-based foods, in moderation. According to the diet theory, this blood type might not be well suited to some of the lectins in soy.

5. Legumes:

- For those with Type B Negative blood, lentils are advised to be consumed in moderation even though they can be a good source of protein and fiber. According to the Blood Type Diet theory, lentil lectins might not be as well-tolerated.

Foods that Could Have a Negative Impact on Blood Type B

1. Almonds:

- Because of lectins and possible adverse effects on digestion, people with Type B Negative blood are frequently advised against consuming peanuts and peanut products.

2. Seeds of Sesame:

- It is advised that people who are Type B Negative limit their intake of sesame seeds and sesame oil. According to the theory, some sesame components might not be well-tolerated.

3. Warm wheat:

- In addition to being cautioned as a problematic protein, buckwheat is also listed among the foods that may negatively affect Type B Negative individuals overall.

4. Chicken Liver:

- Chicken liver, in particular, is noted as a food to avoid for Type B Negative individuals. The theory suggests that proteins in chicken liver may not be well-received by individuals with this blood type.

5. Shellfish:

- Beyond being a troublesome protein, shrimp is also identified as a food that may negatively affect those with

Type B Negative blood. The idea claims that specific components in shellfish may not fit well with this blood type.

CHAPTER 6

Meat and Poultry

To Embrace:

Meat and Poultry to Embrace	Portion Size	Suggested Frequency per Week
Lean Chicken (skinless)	3-4 ounces	3-4 times
Turkey (skinless)	3-4 ounces	3-4 times
Lamb/Mutton (lean cuts)	3-4 ounces	2-3 times
Fish (salmon, mackerel, cod)	4-6 ounces	3-4 times
Trout	4-6 ounces	2-3 times
Halibut	4-6 ounces	2-3 times
Eggs (free-range, omega-3)	2-3 eggs	3-4 times
Tofu	4-6 ounces	2-3 times
Tempeh	4-6 ounces	2-3 times
Lentils (in moderation)	1/2 cup cooked	2-3 times
Black Beans (in moderation)	1/2 cup cooked	2-3 times

To Avoid or Limit:

Meat and Poultry to Avoid or Limit	Portion Size	Suggested Frequency per Week
Chicken (avoid)	-	-
Pork (limit)	3-4 ounces	1-2 times
Processed Meats (sausages, bacon)	Limit	1-2 times
Shellfish (shrimp, crab)	4-6 ounces	1-2 times
Chicken Liver (avoid)	-	-

Diary and Eggs

To Embrace:

Dairy and Eggs	Portion Size	Suggested Frequency per Week
Low-Fat or Skim Milk	1 cup	3-4 times
Yogurt (low-fat, plain)	6 ounces	3-4 times
Goat's Milk Products	-	-
Omega-3 Enriched Eggs	2 eggs	3-4 times

| Cheese (certain varieties) | 1 ounce | 2-3 times |

To Avoid or Limit:

Dairy and Eggs	Portion Size	Suggested Frequency per Week
Full-Fat Milk	1 cup	Limit
Whole Milk Yogurt	6 ounces	Limit
Cheese (certain varieties)	1 ounce	Limit
Ice Cream	1/2 cup	Limit
Processed Cheese	1 ounce	Limit
Blue Cheese	1 ounce	Limit
Cottage Cheese (limit)	1/2 cup	1-2 times
Butter (limit)	1 tablespoon	1-2 times

Seafoods

To Embrace:

Seafoods	Portion Size	Suggested Frequency per Week
Salmon	4-6 ounces	3-4 times
Mackerel	4-6 ounces	3-4 times
Cod	4-6 ounces	3-4 times

Trout	4-6 ounces	2-3 times
Halibut	4-6 ounces	2-3 times
Tuna (in moderation)	4-6 ounces	1-2 times
Sardines	3-4 ounces	1-2 times
Mahi Mahi	4-6 ounces	2-3 times

To Avoid or Limit:

Seafoods	Portion Size	Suggested Frequency per Week
Shrimp	4-6 ounces	1-2 times
Crab	4-6 ounces	1-2 times
Lobster	4-6 ounces	1-2 times
Clams	4-6 ounces	1-2 times
Scallops	4-6 ounces	1-2 times
Octopus (limit)	4-6 ounces	1-2 times
Oysters (limit)	4-6 ounces	1-2 times
Caviar (limit)	1 ounce	1-2 times

Nuts and Seeds

To Embrace

Nuts and Seeds	Portion Size	Suggested Frequency per Week
Almonds	1 ounce	3-4 times
Walnuts	1 ounce	3-4 times
Pine Nuts	1 ounce	2-3 times
Hazelnuts	1 ounce	2-3 times
Flaxseeds	1 tablespoon	3-4 times
Chia Seeds	1 tablespoon	3-4 times
Pumpkin Seeds (pepitas)	1 ounce	3-4 times

To Avoid or Limit:

Nuts and Seeds	Portion Size	Suggested Frequency per Week
Cashews (limit)	1 ounce	1-2 times
Peanuts	1 ounce	Limit
Pistachios (limit)	1 ounce	1-2 times
Sunflower Seeds (limit)	1 ounce	1-2 times
Sesame Seeds (limit)	1 tablespoon	1-2 times
Peanut Butter (limit)	1 tablespoon	1-2 times

| Sunflower Butter (limit) | 1 tablespoon | 1-2 times |

Grains and Cereals

To Embrace:

Grains and Cereals	Portion Size	Suggested Frequency per Week
Quinoa	1/2 cup cooked	3-4 times
Millet	1/2 cup cooked	2-3 times
Oats (steel-cut)	1/2 cup cooked	3-4 times
Brown Rice	1/2 cup cooked	2-3 times
Basmati Rice	1/2 cup cooked	2-3 times
Sprouted Grains (bread)	1 slice	2-3 times

To Avoid or Limit:

Grains and Cereals	Portion Size	Suggested Frequency per Week
Wheat (bread, pasta)	Limit	1-2 times
Buckwheat (limit)	1/2 cup cooked	1-2 times
Corn (limit)	1/2 cup cooked	1-2 times
Barley (limit)	1/2 cup cooked	1-2 times
Rye (limit)	1 slice	1-2 times

Bulgar (limit)	1/2 cup cooked	1-2 times
White Rice (limit)	1/2 cup cooked	1-2 times
Cornflakes (limit)	1 cup	1-2 times

Beverages, Teas, and Coffee

To Embrace:

Beverages, Teas, and Coffee	Portion Size	Suggested Frequency per Week
Green Tea	1-2 cups	Daily
Peppermint Tea	1-2 cups	Daily
Ginger Tea	1-2 cups	Daily
Hibiscus Tea	1-2 cups	Daily
Rooibos Tea	1-2 cups	Daily
Water (hydration)	8-10 cups	Daily

To Avoid or Limit

Beverages, Teas, and Coffee	Portion Size	Suggested Frequency per Week
Black Tea	1-2 cups	1-2 times
Coffee	1 cup	1-2 times
Oolong Tea	1-2 cups	1-2 times
White Tea	1-2 cups	1-2 times
Regular Iced Tea	1 cup	1-2 times

Soda (limit or avoid)	-	-

Fruits

To Embrace

Fruits	Portion Size	Suggested Frequency per Week
Berries (blueberries, strawberries, raspberries)	1 cup	3-4 times
Pineapple	1 cup	2-3 times
Papaya	1 cup	2-3 times
Plums	2 medium	2-3 times
Grapes	1 cup	2-3 times
Cherries	1 cup	2-3 times
Watermelon	1 cup	1-2 times
Figs	2 medium	1-2 times

To Avoid or Limit

Fruits	Portion Size	Suggested Frequency per Week
Oranges	1 medium	Limit
Bananas	1 medium	Limit
Mangoes	1 cup	Limit

Coconut	1/2 cup	Limit
Avocado	1/2 medium	Limit
Persimmons	1 medium	Limit
Pomegranate	1/2 medium	Limit

Vegetables

To Embrace

Vegetables	Portion Size	Suggested Frequency per Week
Spinach	1 cup	3-4 times
Kale	1 cup	3-4 times
Broccoli	1 cup	3-4 times
Swiss Chard	1 cup	2-3 times
Sweet Potato	1 medium	2-3 times
Carrots	1 medium	2-3 times
Beetroot	1 cup	2-3 times
Eggplant	1 cup	2-3 times

To Avoid or Limit

Vegetables	Portion Size	Suggested Frequency per Week
Tomatoes (limit)	1 medium	1-2 times
Corn (limit)	1 cup	1-2 times
Avocado (limit)	1/2 medium	1-2 times

Olives (limit)	10 olives	1-2 times
Brussels Sprouts (limit)	1 cup	1-2 times
Cabbage (limit)	1 cup	1-2 times
Cauliflower (limit)	1 cup	1-2 times

Beans and Legumes

To Embrace

Beans and Legumes	Portion Size	Suggested Frequency per Week
Lentils (in moderation)	1/2 cup cooked	2-3 times
Black Beans (in moderation)	1/2 cup cooked	2-3 times
Navy Beans (in moderation)	1/2 cup cooked	2-3 times
Kidney Beans (in moderation)	1/2 cup cooked	2-3 times
Pinto Beans (in moderation)	1/2 cup cooked	2-3 times
Garbanzo Beans (Chickpeas)	1/2 cup cooked	2-3 times
Adzuki Beans (in moderation)	1/2 cup cooked	2-3 times

To Avoid or Limit

Beans and Legumes	Portion Size	Suggested Frequency per Week
Red Lentils (limit)	1/2 cup cooked	1-2 times
Mung Beans (limit)	1/2 cup cooked	1-2 times
Lima Beans (limit)	1/2 cup cooked	1-2 times
Soybeans (limit)	1/2 cup cooked	1-2 times
Tofu (limit)	4-6 ounces	1-2 times
Tempeh (limit)	4-6 ounces	1-2 times
Black-Eyed Peas (limit)	1/2 cup cooked	1-2 times

Oils and Fats

To Embrace

Oils and Fats	Portion Size	Suggested Frequency per Week
Olive Oil	1 tablespoon	3-4 times
Flaxseed Oil	1 tablespoon	2-3 times
Walnut Oil	1 tablespoon	2-3 times
Ghee (clarified butter)	1 tablespoon	2-3 times
Almond Butter (in moderation)	1 tablespoon	1-2 times
Avocado Oil	1 tablespoon	2-3 times

| Sesame Oil | 1 tablespoon | 1-2 times |

To Avoid or Limit

Oils and Fats	Portion Size	Suggested Frequency per Week
Corn Oil	1 tablespoon	Limit
Soybean Oil	1 tablespoon	Limit
Canola Oil	1 tablespoon	Limit
Peanut Oil	1 tablespoon	Limit
Cottonseed Oil	1 tablespoon	Limit
Sunflower Oil	1 tablespoon	Limit
Margarine (limit)	1 tablespoon	1-2 times

CHAPTER 7

Recipes and How to Prepare Them

10 Breakfast Recipes

1. Breakfast Bowl with Quinoa

- ***Components:***
- Half a cup of cooked quinoa
- berries (strawberries and blueberries)
- One-tspn flaxseed oil
- One tablespoon of finely chopped walnuts
- Honey is optional.

Guidelines:

1. Put the cooked quinoa and berries in a bowl.

2. Sprinkle chopped walnuts on top and drizzle with flaxseed oil.

3. Add honey if you'd like it sweeter.

4. Blend thoroughly and savor!

2. Omelet with Egg and Spinach

Components:

- Two eggs enhanced with omega-3
- a little handful of spinach
- One tablespoon of olive oil
- To taste, add salt and pepper.

Guidelines:

1. In a bowl, beat eggs and add pepper and salt to taste.
2. In a pan with heated olive oil, add the spinach and sauté until it wilts.
3. Over the spinach, pour the beaten eggs.
4. Allow it cool, then fold in half and serve.

3. Bowl of Berry Smoothie

Components:

- One cup of mixed berries (strawberries and blueberries)
- half a cup of yogurt with reduced fat
- One spoonful of chia seeds
- One tablespoon of moderately-sized almond butter

Guidelines:

1. Berries, yogurt, and almond butter should be blended until smooth.

2. Transfer into a bowl and top with chia seeds.

3. Savor this cool smoothie bowl!

4. Pancakes made with sweet potatoes

Components:

- one medium-sized shredded sweet potato
- Two eggs enhanced with omega-3
- One tablespoon of coconut oil
- Cinnamon (not required)

Guidelines:

1. Combine beaten eggs with grated sweet potato.

2. Spoon the mixture into pancakes after heating up some coconut oil in a pan.

3. Cook until both sides are golden brown.

4. If preferred, top with cinnamon and serve.

5. Tomato Salsa with Avocado Toast

Components:

- 1 piece of bread with sprouted grains

- Half a ripe avocado
- One medium tomato, chopped
- One tablespoon of olive oil
- To taste, add salt and pepper.

Guidelines:

1. Toast the bread with sprouted grains.

2. Spread avocado on the toast after mashing it.

3. Combine chopped tomato, olive oil, salt, and pepper in a bowl.

4. Add some tomato salsa to the avocado toast.

6. Pudding with Chia Seeds

Components:

- Two tsp of chia seeds
- half a cup of almond milk
- Half a cup of mixed berries
- One spoonful of honey, if desired

Guidelines:

1. In a jar, combine almond milk and chia seeds.

2. Store in the fridge for several hours or overnight.

3. If preferred, add a drizzle of honey and top with a mixture of berries.

7. Omelet with spinach and feta

Components:

- Two eggs enhanced with omega-3
- a little handful of spinach
- 1/4 cup of feta cheese, crumbled
- One tablespoon of olive oil

Guidelines:

1. In a bowl, beat eggs and season.

2. In olive oil, sauté spinach until it wilts.

3. Cover spinach with beaten eggs and top with feta.

4. Cook, folding, and serving until set.

8. Berry and Walnut Parfait

Components:

- half a cup of yogurt with reduced fat
- 1/4 cup of walnuts, chopped
- Half a cup of mixed berries
- One tablespoon of honey

Guidelines:

1. Arrange berries, walnuts, and yogurt in a glass.

2. Pour some honey in between the layers.

3. Continue until all of the glass is full.

9. Almond milk and millet porridge

Components:

- Half a cup of cooked millet
- half a cup of almond milk
- sliced plums
- One-tspn flaxseed oil

Guidelines:

1. Blend cooked millet with warmed almond milk.

2. Drizzle with flaxseed oil and top with sliced plums.

3. Mix thoroughly and savor.

10. Berry and Greek Yogurt Parfait

Components:	**Guidelines:**
• One cup Greek yogurt (low-fat) • Half a cup of mixed berries • One spoonful of chia seeds • One tablespoon of moderately-sized almond butter	1. Arrange almond butter, chia seeds, berries, and Greek yogurt in a glass. 2. Iterate through the levels. Add one last layer of berries on top.

10 Lunch Recipes

1. Salad with Quinoa and Salmon

Components:

- Salmon fillet, 4-6 ounces
- Half a cup of cooked quinoa
- Various greens
- 1/4 cup chopped cherry tomatoes
- Lemon dressing with olive oil

Guidelines:

1. Bake or grill the fish until it's done.

2. Combine cooked quinoa, cherry tomatoes, and mixed greens.

3. Place the salmon on top of the salad.

4. Add a drizzle of lemon dressing and olive oil.

2. Tofu Stir-Fried with Veggies

Components:

- 4–6 ounces of diced tofu

- mixed veggies, including carrots, bell peppers, and broccoli
- One tablespoon of sesame oil
- Soy sauce or tamarind

Guidelines:

1. Tofu and veggies should be stir-fried in sesame oil.

3. Use soy sauce or tamari to season.

4. Serve with quinoa or brown rice.

3. Bowl of Greek Chicken Salad

Components:

- Grilled chicken breast, 4–6 ounces
- Various greens
- Diced cucumber
- Feta cheese, broken up
- Olives kalamata
- Lemon dressing with olive oil

Guidelines:

After grilling, cut the chicken into strips.

Toss mixed greens with olives, feta, and cucumber.

Add some grilled chicken to the salad.

Add a drizzle of lemon dressing and olive oil.

4. Omelet wrap with spinach and mushrooms

Components:

- Two eggs enhanced with omega-3
- a little handful of spinach
- chopped mushrooms
- Whole-grain tortilla
- Olive oil

Guidelines:

1. Add salt and pepper to the beaten eggs.

2. In olive oil, sauté the spinach and mushrooms.

3. Over the vegetables, pour the beaten eggs and simmer until set.

4. In a whole-grain wrapper, place the omelette.

5. Avocado and Turkey Lettuce Wraps

Components:

- Turkey cutlets
- Lettuce stems
- Sliced avocado
- Sliced tomato
- Mustard (not required)

Guidelines:

1. Place slices of turkey on lettuce leaves.

2. Add the tomato and avocado slices.

3. If desired, drizzle with mustard.

4. Make wraps out of the lettuce leaves.

6. Stir-fried millet and vegetables

Components:

- Half a cup of cooked millet
- Various veggies, including snap peas, bell peppers, and broccoli
- One tablespoon of coconut oil
- Soy sauce or tamarind

Guidelines:

1. Sauté veggies with coconut oil.

2. Toss in the cooked millet.

3. Use soy sauce or tamari to season.

7. Quinoa Bowl with Eggplant and Tomato

<table>
<tr><td>

Components:

- Half a cup of cooked quinoa
- Diced eggplant
- Half a cherry tomato
- Feta cheese, broken up
- Olive oil

</td><td>

Guidelines:

1. Cut eggplant and roast or sauté it until it's soft.

2. Combine the feta, tomatoes, and eggplant with the cooked quinoa.

3. Pour some olive oil over it.

</td></tr>
</table>

8. Salad with Chickpeas and Spinach

<table>
<tr><td>

Components:

- Half a cup of canned, drained chickpeas
- fresh leaves of spinach
- Half a cherry tomato
- Slices of red onion, thinly
- Tahini-lemon dressing

</td><td>

Guidelines:

1. Add the red onion, tomatoes, spinach, and chickpeas.

2. Pour in some lemon-tahini sauce.

</td></tr>
</table>

9. Stuffed bell peppers with lentils and vegetables

<table>
<tr><td>

Components:

- Cut bell peppers in half
- half a cup of cooked lentils
- mixed veggies, including onions, carrots, and zucchini
- Said sauce

</td><td>

Guidelines:

1. Add cooked lentils to a sautéed mixture of mixed veggies.

2. Pack the lentil and veggie mixture inside bell peppers.

3. Bake peppers until they become soft.

</td></tr>
</table>

4. Accompany with a portion of tomato sauce.

10. Walnut and Mackerel Salad

Components:

- Mackerel, grilled, 4–6 ounces
- Various greens
- chopped walnuts
- sliced plums
- dressing with balsamic vinaigrette

Guidelines:

1. Cook the mackerel on the grill.

2. Combine sliced plums and walnuts with mixed leaves.

3. Add some grilled mackerel to the salad.

4. Balsamic vinaigrette dressing should be drizzled on.

Dinner Recipes

1. Stir-fried salmon and asparagus

Components:

- Salmon fillet, 4-6 ounces
- spears of asparagus
- One tablespoon of olive oil
- Soy sauce or tamarind
- minced garlic

Guidelines:

1. Cube the fish and stir-fry it with the asparagus in olive oil.

2. Add soy sauce or tamari and minced garlic.

3. Cook until asparagus is tender and fish is cooked through.

2. Stuffed Bell Peppers with Quinoa

Components:

- Cut bell peppers in half
- Half a cup of cooked quinoa
- Ground chicken or turkey
- Said sauce
- Italian seasonings and herbs

Guidelines:

1. Combine cooked quinoa with ground turkey or chicken that has been brown.

2. Stuff mixture into bell peppers.

3. Add some herbs and tomato sauce over top.

4. Bake peppers until they become soft.

3. Stir-fried Tofu and Vegetables

Components:

- 4–6 ounces of diced tofu
- Various veggies, including snap peas, bell peppers, and broccoli
- One tablespoon of sesame oil
- chopped ginger
- Soy sauce or tamarind

Guidelines:

1. Tofu and veggies should be stir-fried in sesame oil.

2. Add soy sauce or tamari and minced ginger.

3. Sauté the veggies until they are crisp-tender and the tofu turns golden.

4. Buddha Bowl with Millet and Vegetables

Components:

- Half a cup of cooked millet

- Various greens
- Sliced avocado
- Half a cherry tomato
- Drained and canned chickpeas
- dressing with tahini

Guidelines:

1. In a bowl, arrange mixed greens.

2. Add the chickpeas, avocado, tomatoes, and millet over top.

Pour over some tahini dressing.

5. Stuffed Mushrooms with Spinach and Turkey

Components:

- Minced turkey
- cleaned and stem-free mushrooms
- chopped spinach
- Feta cheese, broken up
- Olive oil

Guidelines:

1. Cook minced turkey till browned.

2. Stir in feta and chopped spinach.

3. Once the mushrooms are soft, stuff the caps and bake them.

6. Zoodles with Lemon Garlic Shrimp

Components:

- Peeled and deveined shrimp
- spiralized zucchini to make zoodles
- Lemon extract
- minced garlic
- Olive oil

Guidelines:

1. Garlic powder and shrimp are sautéed in olive oil.

2. Cook the zoodles until they become soft.

3. Before serving, drizzle some lemon juice over it.

7. Curry with chickpeas and vegetables

Components:

- Half a cup of canned, drained chickpeas
- Vegetable mixture (carrots, cauliflower, peas)
- Milk from coconuts
- Curry seasoning
- Grains of brown rice

Guidelines:

1. Cook chickpeas and mixed vegetables in coconut milk.

2. After adding the curry powder, boil the veggies until they are soft.

3. Put on top of brown rice

8. Quinoa with Miso-Glazed Eggplant

Components:

- Sliced eggplant
- Half a cup of cooked quinoa
- paste made with miso
- Soy sauce
- seeds from sesame

Guidelines:

1. Cuts of eggplant can be roasted or grilled till soft.

2. To produce a glaze, combine miso paste and soy sauce.

3. Over the eggplant, drizzle the miso glaze.

4. Place on top of cooked quinoa.

9. Avocado and Mackerel Salad

Components:

- Mackerel, grilled, 4–6 ounces
- Various greens

- Sliced avocado
- Half a cherry tomato
- dressing with balsamic vinaigrette

Guidelines:

1. Cook the mackerel on the grill.

2. On a platter, arrange mixed greens.

3. Add tomatoes, avocado, and mackerel on top.

4. Balsamic vinaigrette dressing should be drizzled on.

10. Stuffed Cabbage Rolls with Mushrooms and Lentils

Components:

- Collard greens
- half a cup of cooked lentils
- chopped mushrooms
- Said sauce
- Italian seasonings and herbs

Guidelines:

1. Sauté the cabbage leaves and reserve.

2. Add chopped mushrooms to cooked lentils.

3. Roll after spooning mixture onto cabbage leaves.

4. Transfer to a baking dish, pour tomato sauce over it, and bake for the desired amount of heat.

Snacks and Appetizers

1. Walnut and Avocado Dip

Components:

- One mature avocado
- 1/4 cup of walnuts, chopped
- Lemon extract
- To taste, add salt and pepper.
- vegetable sticks to dip

Guidelines:

1. Add the chopped walnuts to the mashed avocado.

2. Taste and add salt, pepper, and lemon juice.

3. Accompany with vegetable sticks such as carrots and celery.

2. Berry and Yogurt Parfait Cups

Components:

- One cup Greek yogurt (low-fat)
- Berries in combination (strawberries, blueberries)
- One spoonful of chia seeds
- One tablespoon of moderately-sized almond butter

Guidelines

1. Arrange almond butter, chia seeds, berries, and Greek yogurt in little cups.

2. Iterate through the levels.

3. Keep chilled until you're ready to serve.

3. Hummus and Cucumber Bites

Components:

- Slices of cucumber
- Hummus
- Half a cherry tomato
- Drizzle of olive oil

Guidelines:

1. Spread cucumber slices with hummus.

2. Add cherry tomato halves on top.

3. After adding a little olive oil, serve.

4. Trail Mix Nuts and Berries

Components:

- Almonds
- Cashews
- Pimientos, or pumpkin seeds
- Berries (blueberries, cranberries) dried
- Chips made of dark chocolate (in moderation)

Guidelines:

Combine chocolate chips, walnuts, pumpkin seeds, and dried berries.

Divide into snack-sized bags so you can quickly grab and go.

5. Skewers with Capers

Components:

- rosy tomatoes
- new mozzarella sticks
- Basil foliage
- Drizzle of balsamic glaze

Guidelines:

1. Put basil leaves, mozzarella balls, and cherry tomatoes on little skewers.

2. Before serving, drizzle with balsamic glaze.

6. Edamame Sesame Ginger

Components:

- Edamame legumes
- oil from sesame
- Soy sauce
- chopped ginger

Guidelines:

1. Edamame can be cooked or steamed till soft.

2. Add soy sauce, minced ginger, and sesame oil.

3. Serve as a tasty snack made with edamame.

7. Parfait with Chia Seed Pudding

Components:

- Two tsp of chia seeds
- half a cup of almond milk
- Greek yogurt
- Various berries

Guidelines:

1. Blend almond milk and chia seeds together, then chill until the mixture thickens.

2. Arrange mixed berries and Greek yogurt on top of chia pudding.

3. Iterate through the levels.

8. Roasted lentils

Components:

- Half a cup of canned, drained chickpeas
- Olive oil
- Paprika
- Powdered garlic

Guidelines:

1. Combine garlic powder, paprika, and olive oil with the chickpeas.

2. Roast till crispy in the oven.

3. Let cool before consuming as a snack.

9. Avocado and Sardine Bruschetta

Components:

- pieces of whole-grain baguette
- Mashed avocado
- Sardines with extra virgin olive oil
- Lemon extract
- chopped cherry tomatoes

Guidelines:

1. Toast the slices of baguette.

2. On each slice, spread avocado mash.

3. Add chopped cherry tomatoes, a squeeze of lemon juice, and a sardine on top.

10. Guacamole with pumpkin seeds

Components:

- Mashed avocado
- Toasted pumpkin seeds (pepitas)
- finely sliced red onion
- chopped cilantro
- Lime juice
- Chips with tortillas for dipping

Guidelines:

1. Combine lime juice, red onion, cilantro, and toasted pumpkin seeds with mashed avocado.

2. Accompany with tortilla chips.

Delectable Desserts

1. A parfait with berries and coconut cream

Components:

- Berries in combination (strawberries, blueberries)
- Cream of coconut
- coconut shreds (in moderation)
- Honey is optional.

Guidelines:

1. Arrange the coconut cream and mixed berries in serving cups.

2. If preferred, garnish with shredded coconut and a honey drizzle.

2. Almonds Coated in Dark Chocolate

Components:

- Almonds
- Dark chocolate containing 70% or more cocoa
- sea salt

Guidelines:

In a bowl, melt the dark chocolate.

Almonds are dipped in melted chocolate.

After sprinkling with sea salt, allow them to cool.

3. Walnuts and Cinnamon Apple Bake

Components:

- Sliced apple
- Turnip
- chopped walnuts
- Honey is optional.

Guidelines:

1. Put apple slices in a baking sheet arrangement.

2. Add walnuts that have been chopped and cinnamon.

3. Bake the apples until they are soft.

4. If desired, drizzle with honey.

4. Pudding with Coconut Chia Seeds

Components:

- Two tsp of chia seeds
- half a cup of coconut milk
- Shredded coconut without sugar (in moderation)
- fresh slices of mango

Guidelines:

1. Stir in chia seeds and coconut milk; chill until the mixture thickens.

2. Chia pudding layered with slices of fresh mango.

3. Add some shredded coconut on top.

5. Baked Pears with Cinnamon and Honey

Components:

- Cut pears in half
- Turnip
- chopped pecans
- Honey is optional.

Guidelines:

1. Put the pears cut in half on a baking pan.

2. Add pecans that have been chopped and cinnamon.

3. Bake pears until they are soft.

4. If desired, drizzle with honey.

6. Berries and Honey with Greek Yogurt

Components:

- Greek yogurt with little fat
- Various berries
- Sweetheart
- Pistachios, chopped (in moderation)

Guidelines:

Pour Greek yogurt into dishes for serving.

Add a mixture of berries on top.

After adding a honey drizzle, top with chopped pistachios.

7. Chia Pudding with Pumpkin Spice

Components:

- Two tsp of chia seeds
- half a cup of almond milk
- pureed pumpkin
- Spiced pumpkin
- (Optional) maple syrup

Guidelines:

1. Combine pumpkin puree, almond milk, and chia seeds.

2. If desired, add pumpkin spice and sweeten with maple syrup.

3. Put in the fridge to get it thicker.

8. Popsicles with frozen berries and bananas

Components:

- Diced ripe bananas
- Various berries
- Greek yogurt
- Sweetheart

Guidelines:

1. In popsicle molds, arrange banana slices, mixed berries, and Greek yogurt.

2. Pour some honey in between the layers.

3. Freeze until it solidifies.

9. Avocado with Chocolate Mousse

Components:

- ripe avocado
- powdered cocoa
- Maple syrup.
- extract from vanilla

Guidelines:

1. Avocado, vanilla extract, maple syrup, and cocoa powder should all be blended until smooth.

2. Place in the fridge to cool down before serving.

Components:

- Almond meal
- Eggs
- berries
- Maple syrup.
- icing sugar

Guidelines:

1. Combine the eggs, baking powder, blueberries, maple syrup, and almond flour.

2. Fill muffin tins with batter, then bake until golden.

Smoothies

1. Joyful Berry Smoothie

Components:

- ½ cup mixed berries, including strawberries and blueberries
- half a banana
- half cup of Greek yogurt
- One spoonful of chia seeds
- Almond milk, as required

Guidelines:

1. Smoothly blend the berries, banana, Greek yogurt, and chia seeds.

2. In order to get the right consistency, add almond milk.

3. Savor this smoothie full with antioxidants!

2. Goddess Green Smoothie

Components:

- a little handful of spinach
- half an avocado
- half a cucumber, sliced
- mint leaves that are fresh

- Coconut water, as required

Guidelines:

1. Smoothly blend spinach, avocado, cucumber, and mint.

2. To get the right thickness, add coconut water.

3. Try this nutrient-rich green smoothie to feel refreshed.

3. Tropical Delight with Turmeric

Components:

- half a cup of chunky pineapple
- Half a mango, chopped and skinned
- one-half tsp turmeric powder
- half a cup of nonfat coconut milk
- Cubes of ice

Guidelines:

1. Puree the pineapple, mango, coconut milk, and turmeric until smooth.

2. Mix with the ice cubes once more.

3. Enjoy this delicious tropical turmeric drink!

4. Protein-Rich Almond Butter Drink

Components:

- One spoonful of butter made of almonds
- half a banana
- half cup of Greek yogurt
- half a cup of almond milk
- One-third tsp flaxseed meal

Guidelines:

1. Smoothly blend almond butter, banana, flaxseed meal, Greek yogurt, and almond milk.

2. If necessary, thin the consistency with additional almond milk.

3. Use this high-protein smoothie as fuel.

5. Dream of Cocoa Avocado

Components:

- half an avocado
- One tsp of cocoa powder
- One tablespoon of honey
- Half a cup of low-fat milk (vegan or dairy)
- Cubes of ice

Guidelines:

1. Puree the avocado, milk, honey, and cocoa powder until smooth.

2. Mix with the ice cubes once more.

3. Savor this fantasy of avocados and chocolate!

6. Boost Beet Berry

Components:

- one-half cooked beet, chopped and skinned
- Half a cup of mixed berries
- half cup of Greek yogurt
- One spoonful of chia seeds
- Water (as required)

Guidelines:

1. Puree the cooked beetroot, Greek yogurt, chia seeds, and mixed berries till smooth.

2. To get the right consistency, add water.

3. Savor this colorful, nutrient-dense smoothie.

7. Paradise Smoothie with Papaya

Components:

- half a cup chopped papaya
- half a banana
- half a cup of nonfat coconut milk
- One tablespoon of coconut shreds (in moderation)
- Cubes of ice

Guidelines:

1. Smoothly blend the papaya, banana, coconut milk, and shredded coconut.

2. Mix with the ice cubes once more.

3. Enjoy the papaya paradise smoothie's exotic tastes.

8. Cherry Almond Joy

Components:

- half a cup of pitted cherries
- half a cup of almond milk
- half cup of Greek yogurt
- One spoonful of butter made of almonds
- Cubes of ice

Guidelines:

1. Greek yogurt, almond butter, almond milk, and cherries are blended until smooth.

2. Mix with the ice cubes once more.

3. Savor the delicious fusion of almonds and cherries!

9. Cooler with Mint Melon

Components:

- Half a cup of chopped honeydew melon
- half a cucumber, sliced
- mint leaves that are fresh
- half a cup of coconut water
- Cubes of ice

Guidelines:

1. Mint, cucumber, honeydew melon, and coconut water should all be blended until smooth.

2. Mix with the ice cubes once more.

3. This minty melon cooler will keep you feeling cool!

10. Orange Juice with Carrots and Citrus

Components:

- half an orange, divided and peeled
- 1 1/2 carrots, cut and peeled
- half cup of Greek yogurt
- One tablespoon of honey
- Water (as required)

Guidelines:

1. Smoothly blend orange, carrot, Greek yogurt, and honey.

2. If necessary, dilute the consistency with water.

3. Have a drink of this citrus-rich smoothie!

7-Day Meal Plan

Day 1:

Breakfast: Quinoa Breakfast Bowl with Mixed Berries and Flaxseed Oil

Lunch: Salmon and Asparagus Stir-Fry

Dinner: Baked Pears with Honey and Cinnamon

Day 2:

Breakfast: Green Goddess Smoothie (Spinach, Avocado, Cucumber, Mint)

Lunch Tofu and Vegetable Stir-Fry with Brown Rice

Dinner: Quinoa Stuffed Bell Peppers

Day 3:

Breakfast: Greek Yogurt and Berry Parfait Cups

Lunch: Chickpea and Spinach Salad

Dinner: Tofu and Mushroom Omelette Wrap

Day 4:

Breakfast: Berry Bliss Smoothie

Lunch: Greek Chicken Salad Bowl

Dinner: Mackerel and Walnut Salad

Day 5:

Breakfast: Pumpkin Spice Chia Pudding

Lunch: Lentil and Vegetable Stuffed Bell Peppers

Dinner: Stir-Fried Shrimp with Zoodles

Day 6:

Breakfast: Cocoa Avocado Dream Smoothie

Lunch: Millet and Vegetable Stir-Fry

Dinner: Mushroom and Lentil Stuffed Cabbage Rolls

Day 7:

Breakfast: Almond Flour Blueberry Muffins

Lunch: Turkey and Avocado Lettuce Wraps

Dinner: Miso-Glazed Eggplant with Quinoa

Snacks and Desserts (incorporate as desired throughout the week):

Snacks: Nut and Berry Trail Mix, Cucumber and Hummus Bites

Desserts: Dark Chocolate-Dipped Almonds, Coconut Chia Seed Pudding

CONCLUSION

In conclusion, many have had profound transformations as a result of learning about and adopting the Blood Type B negative diet. By making thoughtful dietary decisions based on blood type, a group of coworkers reported feeling more energized, having better digestion, and feeling better overall. This book acts as a guide, showing the significant influence that individualized diet plans may have on day-to-day living. As these people found out, having the correct diet is a tremendous instrument for realizing our potential and developing a more lively, healthy lifestyle. It's not only about what we eat. I hope that everyone is inspired to maintain long-term health and vigor by my investigation into Blood Type B negative eating.

<u>My Little Request</u>

"Dear valued readers, if you found joy in my book, your five-star rating on Amazon would mean the world to me. Please share your positive thoughts with a heartfelt review. Thank you!"

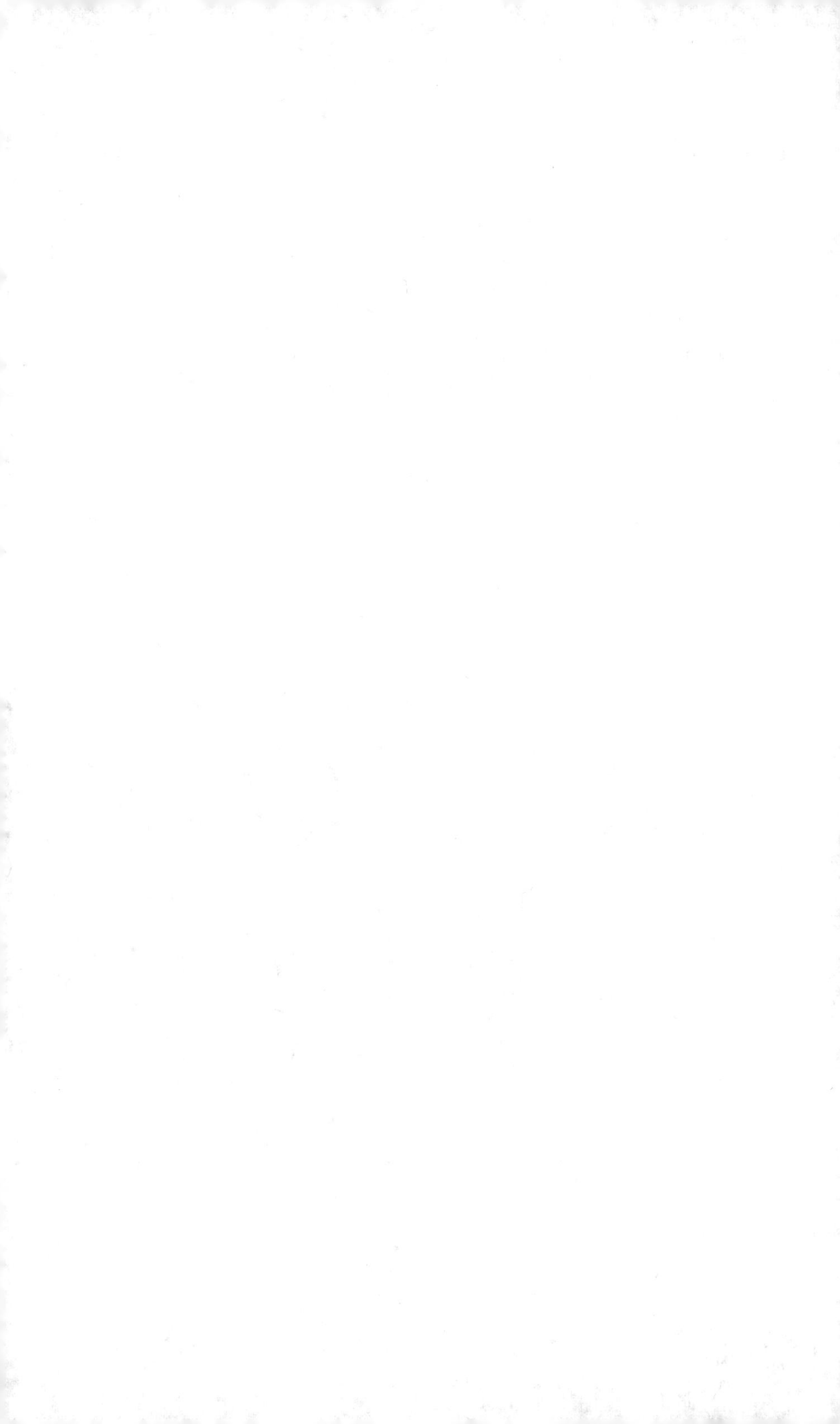